How to Master Menopause

ഇ

Practical Guidance for Dealing with Hot Flashes, Weight Gain, Insomnia, Mood Swings, and Other Menopause Symptoms.

Written by
Vanessa Ford and Danielle Jacobs

Foreword by
Dr. John P. Konhilas, Ph.D

How to Master Menopause: *Practical Guidance for Dealing with Hot Flashes, Weight Gain, Insomnia, Mood Swings, and Other Menopause Symptoms.*

All Rights Reserved © 2020 Vanessa Ford & Danielle Jacobs

www.menolabs.com

ISBN: 978-1629671833

Library of Congress Control Number: Pending

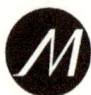

ATTENTION CORPORATIONS, UNIVERSITIES, COLLEGES, AND PROFESSIONAL ORGANIZATIONS

Quantity discounts are available on bulk purchases of this book for educational or gift purposes. Special editions or book excerpts can also be created to fit specific needs.

Visit menolabs.com for more information.

Rev 7.14

Table of Contents

୫୦

Menopause is a natural transition, but it can bring with it significant health impacts that directly affect diseases a woman may face. I believe the microbiome affords us the opportunity to attack the symptoms associated with menopause at the root cause.

୫୦

Foreword

by
Dr. John P. Konhilas, Ph.D

You may be wondering, "why is a 50-year-old male scientist studying menopause?" I am not female. I don't identify as female. I will never experience what it is like to be female or experience menopause. The answer to this question boils down to this: I love thinking about science. My drive and natural curiosity have always encouraged me to pursue the most interesting and impactful science using relevant and appropriate tools. Menopause is one of the most important areas of scientific research that we can study for two primary reasons.

These two facts changed the way I do science and drove me to focus on menopause:

1. Menopause is a condition that every woman will experience. One hundred percent of women who live long enough will go through menopause.
2. Since 1984, more women than men have died from cardiovascular disease. . . and very few people are studying why.

Now, the first statement also includes women who have had their ovaries surgically removed. The second statement most likely comes as a shock to the general public, and especially to women. If we examine the data more closely, we know that women who are diagnosed with heart failure experience worsening heart failure more rapidly than men.

Women over the age of 50 experience worsening heart failure than women under 50. This timeframe closely aligns with the transition from perimenopause to menopause. While the medical and scientific community acknowledge this age-specific presentation of heart failure in women, the correlation with menopausal transition has not.

A very astute physician recognizes that estrogen loss due to the natural transition of menopause masks cardiovascular disease symptoms or underlies cardiovascular disease symptoms that are atypical in comparison to men. For example, over 50% of women present with symptoms of heart failure where their hearts can eject blood to the body normally. The reason why they have heart failure symptoms is that their hearts cannot relax normally. This symptom of heart failure with preserved ejection fraction is present in women twice as often than in men. Why? I can spend pages describing why and describing heart disease differences between men and women, but this problem runs much deeper and is more profound than just sex-differences in cardiovascular disease.

Women Have Been Left Out of Scientific Research for Far Too Long.

Over the last 50 years, females have largely been excluded from experimental designs primarily because females are "too variable." Can you guess why?

The "variability" claim from research organizations is that menstruation and a monthly hormonal cycle make women too variable for many studies. To this day, women continue to be under-represented in clinical trials of all types and, if included, are typically compared to men. I will come back to this point about comparing men to women in a moment.

In response to the sex bias in 2016, the Office of Women's Health Research at the National Institutes of Health mandated studies to require both males and females in preclinical science. In fact, the Office of Women's Health Research went so far as to provide supplemental funding to those individuals with NIH (National Institute of Health) grants to include females in their study design.

When we reached out to the Office of Women's Health Research to have a special funding mechanism for those of us already doing studies exclusively in females, these requests were met by silence. I am amazed and dumbfounded that only within the last four years has there been an acknowledgment of early attempts to provide mechanisms to increase the visibility of females in scientific research.

The Differences Between Men and Women Are Greater Than We Think.

Because the scientific community can now perform large scale genetic analysis, comparisons between men and women using these techniques have been completed. Men and women are about 98.5% genetically similar.

This may seem like men and women are very similar genetically. They are not. If we refer back to the basic principle above that females are "too variable", we are better off comparing men to male chimps because male chimps are as genetically similar (98.5%) to men as men are to women.

Let me repeat that. A human man is as genetically similar to a male chimp as he is to a human woman.

In my opinion, there is no reason to "include" females in research. We need to study women independently of men. Women experience transitions that greatly impact their health. We can use the variability of women to better study disease than we can in men. Imagine if a certain disease was discovered and had a disease penetrance that impacts a single population at a rate of 100%. Imagine that population was only men. How would the scientific community react?

Now, menopause is not a disease. It is a natural part of a woman's life. Menopause has 100% penetrance. Menopause impacts or will impact over half the world's population. Why do we not have a national or international effort to study this? I wrote a grant a few years ago focusing on the impact of menopause and the microbiome on health outcomes in females using a very unique model of menopause developed at the University of Arizona. It was the worst scored grant I ever received, not well received by the community. The critique was a blow to my confidence as a scientist and as a human being who wants to understand menopause. Then, I read a single statement from a 7-page critique that changed my life. The critique stated that I should be "using males as a control in the study on menopause."

I can't even begin to comment on how absolutely ridiculous and insulting that statement is. That statement demonstrates an ignorance that embarrasses the scientific community. Yet, this is how a large portion of the scientific community views this topic.

I will never call menopause a disease. Menopause is a natural transition, but it can bring with it significant health impacts that directly affect diseases a woman may face. I believe the microbiome affords us the opportunity to attack the symptoms associated with menopause at the root cause. By reducing those symptoms and improving the health outcomes for women, we can impact one of the most universal chapters in women's lives.

ॐ

Menopause is not a disease, illness, or condition. Menopause is a natural, biological transition that gets your body from one stage to the next.

ॐ

Introduction - Hi, There! Have You Met Menopause?

What do you think of when you hear the word "menopause"? You might think of the horror stories of hot flashes you've heard from friends. You might think of the rapid accumulation of fine lines and wrinkles. Or, you might wonder how many cheesecakes *The Golden Girls* consumed on a daily basis and if you'll have the same craving when menopause strikes.

Whether you're preparing for menopause, already in menopause, or wishing you had known more when the time came, every woman can feel a bit daunted

by her menopausal journey. Every woman experiences those biological milestones differently from pubescence to pregnancy. In this guide, we hope to provide you with the knowledge you need to best prepare yourself for the challenges you may face in your menopause journey.

What We Think About Menopause Is Wrong.

We often discuss menopause in a very negative way. When we attach a negative value to something, we convince our brains that it's something that should be feared or avoided. Well, you're not going to be able to avoid menopause, but that doesn't mean you should be scared of it. Menopause is not a disease, illness, or condition. Menopause is a natural, biological transition that gets your body from one stage to the next.

If that's true, then why do we perpetuate this idea that menopause is a phase of life that diminishes our value as women, changes us fundamentally as people, and ruins our relationships with others? The truth is, our understanding of menopause has only really been looked into over the last 150 years. This doesn't just encompass the scientific breakthroughs we've had, this applies largely to how we've publicized and propagandized biased and skewed opinions on the subject.

The History of Menopause in Western Society.

Menopause has been a topic of interest for thousands of years. Aristotle himself even studied the subject with great curiosity. That being said, menopause was never really a topic of discussion that the general public engaged in. It was mostly discussed among the elite physicians, who were all male. The variety of opinions they had on the subject were astounding, and in some cases, terrifying.

The Influence of Men: The Victorian Era

From the 1800s on, the discussion surrounding menopause became increasingly biased. The perspective was not from the point of view of the woman, it was from the point of view of the man. Men were largely the only ones practicing medicine, although the first female medical student in the United States graduated college in 1849. Since male physicians were the ones with the most influence during these times, they also had the most influence on how information on women's health (and menopause) were conveyed to the public.

Many people think that propaganda was used largely for wartime, but throughout history, people have propagandized everything from food, to race, to gender, and medicine. Physicians would often publish advertisements in their local paper claiming they could help eliminate menopausal symptoms in women by curing their "hysteria", what they believed to be the source of many female health concerns regardless of age.

English physician Isaac Baker Brown claimed that he could cure female hysteria and all other conditions that stemmed from it, by performing a very specific surgery. According to Brown, menopause and emotional mood swings during periods were caused by female hysteria, and the clitoris was the source of this hysteria. His solution to this problem was to surgically remove the clitoris. Clitorodectomies, which are still practiced to some extent in parts of the world, became a fairly popular form of treatment for a time. However, Brown had performed these surgeries on patients without their knowledge or consent. This practice later became criminalized in England, but some physicians still believed it was a valid form of treatment for women.

Linking Menopause to Femininity: The Early 20th Century

Another phenomenon that happened in western culture, was the development of the concept called, "The Death of the Woman." This concept linked female sexuality, desire, and attraction to the loss of characteristics that women exhibited in their youth. This included physical attributes like youthful, glowing skin but it also included physiological attributes like sexual arousal. Once men began to notice the shift in women's moods, sexual performance, and so on, this marked the transition from woman to crone, hence the phrase, the death of the woman. Medical advertisements during this era were focused on getting women back to exhibiting youthful responses. Health, as well as physical and mental well-being, were not marketed. Instead, changes in personality were marketed.

How Western and Eastern Cultures Differ

While the western perspective on menopause has largely been a negative one, there are other cultures around the world that look at it in a more positive light. In Chinese culture, menopause is often referred to as "the second spring." The second spring is a positive transition. It marks the time when a woman should turn from spending the majority of her energy on nurturing others inward and instead, spend it nurturing herself. Once women reach

this transition, they achieve a heightened sense of wisdom and confidence. While menopausal symptoms remain the same no matter where in the world you are, Chinese culture emphasizes the need to nurture the body and the mind during this phase of life and use it as a way to achieve longevity and lasting inner peace. Having a positive value attached to menopause helps women reap positive benefits to their health as they continue to age.

Getting Comfortable With Your Menopause.

Society's perceptions of a topic cannot change without the spearheading of the individual's thoughts on the matter. Getting comfortable with menopause begins with you.

When it comes to changing the conversation about menopause, there are a few things that you should understand as an individual, and especially as a woman.

1. **Every woman's menopausal experience is different.** Not every woman will experience the same symptoms, have the struggles, or receive the same treatments. Your experience is unique to you.

2. **Menopause is all about navigating the relationship between you and your body.** Learning to listen to your body is tough, but it's necessary during menopause. If something doesn't feel right, make a note of it and find ways to help solve the problem.

3. **Knowledge is key, so talk to your doctor.** We're still learning a lot about menopause and menopausal treatments, and it's impossible for one person to retain all of that information and keep up to date when it's not their job. Talking to your doctor about your concerns, questions, or just general curiosity can help you better understand what you can expect from your menopausal experiences and help you feel better prepared to deal with the more challenging aspects of it.

4. **Talking about it is as important as treating it.** A conversation needs two things, a talker and a listener. Talking about your experiences, struggles, and needs with others can help break down some of the barriers between you and your loved ones. Talk to your friends, family, partners, and other women who are going through similar experiences.

We realize how hard it can be for women to feel comfortable talking about their menopausal concerns with their doctors, friends, and romantic partners. Don't be afraid to start off small and take baby steps. If you're not comfortable talking about specific problem areas, address your other concerns first. That way you can get used to the process.

What Questions Should You Be Asking Your Doctor?

You might be wondering where you should start when talking to your doctor about menopause. With so many issues to discuss, it can be hard to know what you should prioritize in those 30-minute appointments. While you can address all of your concerns with your doctor over the course of a series of appointments, it's important to remember to get the basics done and out of the way first. Here are some of the basics you should cover on your first appointment:

1. What are the most common menopausal symptoms you help your patients with?
2. What methods have worked best for your patients in the past?
3. Of those methods, which do you think will work well for me?
4. Which methods do you think I should stay away from?
5. What lifestyle changes would you recommend I make now given what we've discussed?
6. What do you think I should keep in mind as we go through the treatment process down the line?

If you keep these six questions in mind on your first visit to the doctor, you'll be in a much better position to work with them on a treatment plan that works well for you.

What Research Is Out There?

We've talked about changing the conversation about menopause, the history behind menopause research, and how you can work with your doctor to go about treating it. But what do we really know about menopause when it comes to the research side of things? After all, we've only just begun to treat research into menopause as a worthwhile pursuit.

Even in today's society we're making incredible strides in researching menopause and related topics. While there continue to be challenges in scientific research, the amount of new information we have on the effects and potential treatments for menopause is staggering and continuing to grow. So, what have we really found out?

Research into Probiotics

One of the most interesting areas of study is the research into the relationship between menopausal processes and probiotics. Many women are turning away from standard hormone replacement therapy (HRT) treatment options and searching for other kinds of treatment. Research into the use of probiotics as a way to help alleviate certain menopausal symptoms have turned up some fascinating results and ideas.

What Are Probiotics?

Probiotics are microorganisms, bacteria, that can provide health benefits to the body. Probiotics travel through the digestive system and help the body extract and metabolize nutrients from food and other sources. Having enough healthy bacteria can help your body better regulate other systems which could potentially prevent you from developing illnesses, help you maintain a healthy weight, and help improve hormone regulation.

How Can They Help?

There's a partnership between two major systems that helps regulate the overall health of the human body. It's called the gut-brain axis. The gut-brain axis is the connection between the gut (your stomach and gastrointestinal tract) and the brain. Both the gut and the brain send and receive information that is then used to regulate other processes in the body. By taking in nutrients in the gut, your body metabolizes it through the lining of your intestines and sends it through the bloodstream to be used to regulate other areas of the body. This relationship between the brain and the gut helps keep the systems of your body health.

What Now?

How can probiotics help alleviate some of your menopausal symptoms? What symptoms could even be affected by the use of probiotic supplements? We're here to help you out. In this book we'll look at six of the most common menopausal symptoms and break them down. We'll look into the relationship between estrogen and other systems in your body. We'll discuss how lifestyle changes can help alleviate symptoms. We'll even talk about how to better communicate your needs and struggles with the important people in your life, your doctor, your friends, and your family. Not only that, we'll take a look at what probiotics could help you alleviate specific symptoms and help you understand some of the science behind it.

৶

About 75% of women experience hot flashes during menopause and more than 80% of menopausal women will experience hot flashes for up to 2 years.

৶

Chapter 1 - Hot Flashes

Hot flashes are the most common symptom of menopause, and among the most inconvenient to experience. Described as a sudden rise in body temperature, having a hot flash is like having your own mini summer heat wave just waiting to come out and surprise you. About 75% of women experience hot flashes during menopause and more than 80% of menopausal women will experience hot flashes for up to 2 years.

Of course, every woman will experience hot flashes differently. Some women may have hot flashes that last up to 10 minutes or happen 20 times in a single day.

Vanessa's Story

Before I learned how probiotics could help me, one of my most annoying menopause symptoms was night sweats, which are basically just hot flashes that happen while you're trying to sleep.

At first, I didn't attribute them to menopause. I live in the desert, so sweating and feeling overly warm is pretty common, especially in the summer. But after I discovered it might be perimenopause causing my night-time sweat sessions (see the chapter about changing periods for the story on that!) I found there were steps I could take to control them.

Taking charge of my night sweats has made me feel much more in control of my body. I'm sleeping better, and I am not exhausted throughout the day. The best part is that I learned how to control my night-time hot flashes *before* they had a chance to visit me during the day, and for that, I am incredibly grateful.

How Do Hot Flashes Happen?

Menopause occurs when the primary sex hormones, estrogen and progesterone, begin to decrease. When the production rate of these hormones drops, other systems in the body are affected, especially the brain. You might be wondering, what does the brain have to do with hot flashes?

Internal body temperature is controlled by a part of the brain called the hypothalamus. When estrogen decreases, the hypothalamus becomes more sensitive to changes in temperature. When your brain thinks that your body is becoming too warm, it triggers a surge of heat that's meant to release sweat onto your skin and cool you down. Additionally, estrogen helps regulate the opening and closing of blood vessels, especially near the skin. So when estrogen decreases, these blood vessels swell and cause more heat to be carried to the surface.

Combine these two processes and the result is a sweaty, uncomfortable hot flash.

What Can I Do to Treat Them?

Hot flashes are caused by drops in hormones that make your brain go a little wonky, so what can you do to treat them? Some women may not be able to get rid of hot flashes completely during their menopausal years. However, you can help lower their intensity and their frequency by adjusting three factors in your daily life: diet, exercise, and medication.

Diet

Remember the saying, "you are what you eat?" Well, in this case, it's actually fairly accurate. Eating certain foods might have an effect on how your body regulates its internal temperature.

As we know, drops in estrogen are what cause hot flashes to occur. How can you alter an estrogen imbalance through food? There are certain foods that are high in compounds called phytoestrogens. Phytoestrogens are estrogens that occur naturally in plants like legumes, seeds, soybeans, berries, and many more. Consuming foods with phytoestrogens can help rebalance your hormone levels and keep your hypothalamus from being tricked into thinking it's too warm. There are foods high in phytoestrogens that you should be thinking about incorporating into your diet.

Foods to Eat
- Soy products, like soymilk, tofu, tempeh
- Seeds, like flax seeds and sesame seeds
- Whole grains, like wheat, barley, oats, rice, and lentils
- Berries, like strawberries, cranberries, and raspberries

Foods that are high in phytoestrogens are foods on the pros side of the list. You should also be aware of foods that are on the cons side of the list. Foods that tend to raise internal body temperature, like caffeine, alcohol, and spicy foods, should be avoided to reduce the intensity of hot flashes.

Foods to Avoid
- Large quantities of alcohol (try to limit yourself to one glass of wine or a light beer)
- Caffeinated beverages (coffee and strong teas should be drunk in small amounts)

- High-salt foods (chips, fries, smoked and cured meats)
- Spicy foods (hot peppers like jalapenos, habaneros, and strong chilis)

Another way to adjust your diet to help alleviate hot flashes, is through a moderate protein, low carb, and high good fat diet. How can adjusting these three areas of your diet help reduce the intensity of hot flashes?

Reduced body fat, as a result of adjustments to these areas, showed a variety of health improvements like lower blood pressure, reduced levels of blood lipids like cholesterol and triglycerides, and decreased body temperature.

By adhering to this low-carb, moderate protein, high good fat diet, there was an overall reduction in levels of certain metabolic mediators, hormones that play a role in regulating metabolism. These metabolic mediators include insulin, leptin, glucose, triglycerides, and the thyroid hormone triiodothyronine (T3). Triiodothyronine affects multiple processes in the body, most importantly body temperature and heart rate. By reducing levels of T3, body temperature begins to decrease, which could result in lowering the intensity of hot flashes.

Exercise

Although it may seem counterintuitive, exercise can actually help reduce the frequency of hot flashes, especially if you do it on a regular basis. Now, we know what you're thinking, how does exercise prevent hot flashes? Wouldn't that mean you're getting your body temperature up? Well, yes, exercise does get your body temperature up, but it also starts the natural perspiration process.

Hot flashes only occur when your hypothalamus registers a false increase in body temperature. Exercise bypasses this false trigger and causes your body to produce sweat naturally and throughout the entire body, not just in localized areas.

Have you ever noticed how certain areas of your body are affected more than others during a hot flash? Can you remember where you felt the most heat? Women of menopausal age will typically experience localized areas of heat in the head, neck, upper chest, shoulders, and arms during a hot flash. When you exercise, heat is dispersed throughout your entire body, not just in localized areas. When this happens, your hypothalamus will signal for your skin to release sweat everywhere in an effort to cool down the whole body. The frequency of hot flashes decreases, because the body doesn't need to cool itself down a second time.

We know that exercise helps reduce the frequency of hot flashes, but what kinds of exercise have the biggest impact? The general rule of thumb is, the intense workout produces the strongest results. Now, by no means are we suggesting you go out and participate in a triathlon right out of the gate. We're advocating for healthy exercise, not insanity. However, engaging in moderate to vigorous exercise tailored to your individual needs can be a lifesaver, literally.

What exercises are best for you will depend on a few factors.

1. How often do you exercise now?
1. Regularly
2. Occasionally
3. Never

2. Do you have any underlying health conditions: respiratory issues (asthma), joint issues, muscle issues, etc.?
   1. Yes
   2. No

3. Do you have any past injuries or surgeries you've recovered from?
   1. Yes
   2. No

Keeping your answers to these questions in mind, take a look at these different exercise routines and decide which one you think is right for you. Ask a doctor or a physical therapist for professional advice before you make any major decisions.

For Women With:

- Regular exercise routines
- No underlying health conditions
- No past injuries or surgeries

You're in a better position to engage in more vigorous workouts, but remember to start off slow and build your way up. High cardio workouts and muscle-focused exercises are going to be better options for you.

Try out exercises like:

- Running/Jogging
- Weight lifting
- Swimming
- Intermediate/Advanced Pilates

For Women With:

- Occasional exercise routines
- Some to no underlying health conditions
- Past injuries and surgeries

If your current exercise routine is once every few days or 1-2 times a week, and your exercise routine is more moderate (like yoga or 15-20 minute aerobics exercises), then you may want to adjust certain elements of your workout routine to better reflect your needs.

You can adjust your exercise routine in any number of ways. You can:

- Extend your workout time: Instead of 20 minute workouts, try 30 minute workouts or even an hour.
- Focus on increasing your cardio steadily: Upgrade from walking to jogging, start using resistance bands for building up muscle.
- Keep impact exercises light or moderate for joint problems: Don't do 50 jumping jacks if your knees bother you. Instead, tailor your workout routine to put less pressure on your joints (floor exercises tend to be best for this).

For Women With:

- No exercise routine
- Underlying health conditions
- Past injuries or surgeries

If this list describes your current exercise situation, don't be embarrassed. A lot of women have difficulty keeping up an exercise routine. Whether you have a busy career, a busy home life, or an active life in your community, it may be a real struggle to find time for yourself. That's okay! You don't have to run a marathon to improve your health. You can do it in other smaller, easier ways.

Start with:

- Introducing small bursts of daily workouts into your routine: 15 minutes of exercise everyday, no matter how small can make a big difference in how you feel.
- Increasing your cardio: Just taking a 10 minute walk around the block can boost your cardio. Remember increasing your body temperature through exercise can lower the number of hot flashes you experience in a given day.
- Shift your focus to your core: If you can't participate in running or jogging due to joint problems, you can easily increase your cardio regimen through core exercises (crunches, flutter kicks, modified leg lifts). The more you engage your diaphragm through heavy breathing the higher your body temperature will be.

Probiotic Supplements

Of course, changes to your diet and exercise may only go so far for you. The menopausal experience is different for every woman, and not every woman can solve her hot flashes as easily. When diet and exercise are not enough to help ease hot flashes, what other options are out there for you? Research on how probiotic supplements can be used to treat menopausal symptoms has produced some surprising results.

What are probiotic supplements?
Probiotics are microorganisms that are introduced to the body, whether through food or other sources, that provide health benefits. If you've ever taken a pill for digestion support or regularity, you've taken a probiotic. If you've ever eaten yogurt, you've consumed a probiotic. So, if probiotic supplements are used for gut regularity, how can they help treat your hot flashes?

The Power of the Microbiome
The microbiome is the ecosystem of microorganisms that live inside the body. When these microorganisms are healthy, they help keep our body healthy. How do they do this? The microbiome is connected to the body through something called the gut-brain axis. The gut-brain axis is the connection between the brain and the digestive system. Through this connection the gut and the

brain send and receive nutrients and nerve signals in a continuous loop.

What Probiotics Can Reduce Hot Flashes?

The term probiotics specifically refers to bacterial strains meant to help balance bacterial cultures that live in the body naturally. However, oftentimes these bacterial strains are paired with plant compounds that can provide them with specific nutrients to have greater effects on the body. So what plant compounds can help reduce hot flashes?

Red Clover
Red clover is a type of legume that possesses substances known as isoflavones. Isoflavones are phytoestrogens, plant compounds that simulate the role of estrogen in women.

There are two major isoflavones in red clover, Biochanin A and Formononetin. When combined, both of these isoflavones help rebalance hormones responsible for regulating body temperature.

Milk Thistle

Another botanical ingredient, Milk Thistle extract can be used to treat hot flashes when combined with a probiotic. Milk Thistle can help improve liver function. You may be asking, why is this important to treating hot flashes? The liver is responsible for helping process and regulate hormones throughout the body. During menopause, the drop in estrogen causes a negative impact on liver function, making it more difficult for the liver to process hormones that regulate other areas of the body. This includes the hormones responsible for regulating body temperature. Taking milk thistle extract can help improve liver function and help regulate body temperature by processing those hormones more efficiently.

ॐ

Understanding how your sex drive changes during menopause is the first step to overcoming sexual health problems.

ॐ

Chapter 2 - Low Sex Drive

Let's be honest, how many of you want to skip this chapter entirely out of sheer embarrassment and discomfort? You may not want to admit or talk about it, but the fact is, your sex drive will lower as you progress into menopause. While it may be an uncomfortable subject to talk about with your partner and your doctor, discussing your sexual health concerns can help you maintain a safe, healthy, and active sex life well into the later years of your life.

Of course, finding the courage to talk about such a sensitive issue is easier said than done. A series of surveys of women of midlife ages, primarily in their 50s, found that less than 1/3 of women discuss sexual issues with their healthcare providers. As a result, many women don't get the care and advice they need to continue having a healthy and active sex life. This can cause, not only a number of health problems, but it can also create strain between women and their partners.

Understanding how your sex drive changes during menopause is the first step to overcoming sexual health problems. Once you understand how menopause affects libido, you can turn your attention to addressing your individual health concerns and find solutions that both you and your partner can participate in.

Vanessa's Story

I've spoken with hundreds of women about their menopause experiences, and so many of them have told me about their difficulties maintaining a healthy sex life and while I haven't had this particular menopause symptom myself, women who are going through this should know that they are most definitely not alone!

When I talk to women who tell me about how they cope with this symptom, the first thing they tell me is that they educated themselves, and used that education to make health decision that would improve their sex lives.

Sexual function and desire are really complex, both biologically and emotionally. The best way to determine the root cause of your low sex drive is to research potential causes, and then involve your health care provider in crafting a plan to address them. I hope the information in this chapter will be help you take the first step toward a better sex life.

A Closer Look at Low Libido

Low libido is one of the more common symptoms of menopause, and not all women will experience it in the same way. Some may feel a decrease in their sex drive more rapidly than others. Some women may feel a sudden increase in their sex drive before the drop in hormones causes it to lower and plateau. For many women, it may fluctuate based on changes in their menstrual cycle. How can one symptom have so many varieties?

Sexual arousal is largely dictated by estrogen, with the help of a few other hormones. When estrogen levels begin to deplete, they affect your body's reaction to sexual stimulus and impact arousal.

Estrogen helps regulate blood flow to the vagina. When a woman becomes aroused, the body prepares itself for sexual activity by sending a rush of blood to the vagina. This helps keep the lining of the vaginal canal thick and helps promote the release of natural lubricants that protect the vagina from the irritation of friction.

A drop in estrogen will lower the body's ability to send blood flow

to the vagina as quickly. The lining of the vaginal canal will become shorter and thinner. The vagina won't be able to produce as much natural lubricant to coat the inner lining, causing it to feel dry, uncomfortable, and increase pain and sensitivity during penetrative sex.

Vaginal Dryness and Vaginal Atrophy

The passage above describes two intertwined conditions, vaginal dryness and vaginal atrophy. Vaginal dryness is, just as it sounds, the drying out of the vaginal lining. When natural lubricants cannot be produced, the lining of the vagina becomes thinner and shorter, as it doesn't have the moisture to help it expand. If vaginal dryness becomes severe enough, it can cause vaginal atrophy, which is an extreme thinning of the vaginal lining. Women with vaginal atrophy will often cite experiencing intense pain and discomfort when they engage in penetrative sexual activities.

How to Address Sexual Health Concerns

Discussing sexual health problems is never easy. Talking about sex and sexual health to friends and family can be uncomfortable enough. Talking about it with a doctor, who may or may not be a complete stranger to you, is even more uncomfortable. We get it. It's awkward and embarrassing. It's normal to feel these things, but when your apprehension to talk about it impacts your health, that's when the more difficult problems arise. Your sexual health is just as important as your heart health, immune health, and mental health. Treat it with the same attention.

If you're not sure where to start when it comes to being open about your sexual health concerns, here are some things to keep in mind.

Talking to Your Doctor

It can be awkward talking to a complete stranger about your sexual health problems. To make the experience seem less embarrassing, build a rapport with your doctor. No matter who you choose to see, ultimately a doctor's goal is to help you address your health concerns and get you feeling better. Still, we understand that talking about intimate subjects can be uncomfortable with someone outside of your close friends or family. Build a relationship with your doctor. Build trust, crack a few jokes. If you're not ready to talk about sexual health problems right out of the gate, address other health concerns first as a way to prepare yourself for when you are ready to talk about it.

Start off small. Talk about your concerns over your hot flashes or irregular periods. Then build your way up to talking about things like heart health. When you feel you and your doctor have built up enough of a rapport, talk about your sexual health concerns. You don't have to dive headfirst into anything you don't feel comfortable discussing. You can wait until you're ready to talk about it, just don't wait too long. Above all, remember that your doctor is there to help you out. You're not wasting their time talking about your sexual health problems. They are ready and willing to help you tackle any problem.

Talking to Your Partner

Let's suppose that you've gotten comfortable talking to your doctor about your sexual health concerns. It may still be difficult to talk about these concerns with your partner. Every relationship is different and every couple handles intimacy in a different way. Some couples feel very comfortable talking about their sex lives with each other. Some couples may only feel comfortable talking about certain things with one another. Some couples may not feel like talking about intimate matters with each other at all.

Feeling apprehensive to talk about sex and sexual needs is normal, but if it prevents you from enjoying your sex life, then it becomes a real problem. It can cause tension between couples. It can strain relationships, and it can affect the mental health of both you and your partner.

If you're not sure where to start when you decide to have that conversation, what should you do?

Be Prepared

Talking to your partner about your sexual health problems in mid-life will require some explanation. You can't expect your partner to know everything about how estrogen affects the reproductive system or what happens to the vagina during arousal. Take this time to educate them a bit on what's going on inside your

body. Having some of this knowledge will help them better understand what you're going through and how they can help you solve some of these problems.

Be Relaxed

One of the biggest reasons women refuse to talk about their sexual health problems with their partners is anxiety. Women in heterosexual partnerships tend to have higher anxiety talking about their sexual needs out of fear of being judged or misunderstood. Oftentimes, men and women feel a sense

of disparity when it comes to expressing sexual needs or desires. This may cause them to withhold information out of fear of being ridiculed. Don't let this anxiety prevent you from sharing information with one another.

If you feel relaxed, chances are your partner will feel relaxed, too.

Be Understanding

Your partner may feel just as equally uncomfortable with this conversation as you do. If they seem hesitant to talk about it or they're uncomfortable with discussing details, don't let that get you down. It's not unusual for couples to feel initially awkward about the subject. Be patient and remind them that you're in this together.

What Can You Do to Tackle Sexual Problems?

Sexual health problems in midlife don't have to be an uphill battle. You can find ways to help improve and maintain better sexual health. Whether through experimentation or medicinal treatments, there are a variety of options available to you. So, where should you start?

Solutions in the Bedroom

Lubricants

Vaginal dryness can be uncomfortable, both in general and during sex. When natural lubricant isn't produced as quickly, what can you do to help lower the intensity of friction during sex and keep the vaginal lining from becoming too thin? There are plenty of lubricant products on the market that can help provide you some relief before sex. Look for water-based lubricants to use, not only are they more comfortable but they also don't wear down latex in condoms which you may or may not be using. Additionally, avoid lubricants with glycerin in them, as some women are more prone to developing yeast infections after using.

Foreplay

For many couples out there who engage in sexual activities regularly, foreplay may not seem like a new concept. However, more often than not, couples may not be engaging in enough foreplay before sex. Foreplay can help women's bodies have enough time to prepare itself for sex. It may take longer for blood to flow to the vagina, in which case extending your foreplay time may help your body produce the natural lubricant it requires.

Perhaps you and your partner engage in foreplay regularly but you find the same things aren't working as much as they did before. Try out new things. Whether it's new techniques, new speeds, or new ideas in general, you can find new ways to help you achieve arousal.

Experimentation

Experimentation can go beyond foreplay. Perhaps you and your partner were not very experimental in the past when it came to your sex life, and now you're curious to venture into unexplored territory. Encourage experimentation in one another. It can be beneficial to both you and your partner. Experiment with fantasies, role playing, and sensory play. If you end up finding something that works for both you and your partner, then incorporate it.

Meditation / Mindfulness

Sexual meditation or sexual mindfulness, as it's more commonly referred to, may sound strange at the start, but it's actually been helping women everywhere to get more in tune with their bodies as they change. Sexual meditation is all about establishing a better connection between the mind and the body. Mentality is just as important as physical chemistry when it comes to sex. For many women who are experiencing noticeable changes in their bodies, this can have a significant impact on how they view their bodies during sex.

Having a positive perception about your body can impact how sexy you feel in front of your partner and should be taken into account when discussing your sex life. Sexual mindfulness is all about helping you to feel more comfortable with your body and to be better attuned to it. Focusing on how your body reacts to certain conditions or stimuli can help you better understand what your body needs. Do a little digging into sexual meditation techniques, try them out, and see if they can help you feel more connected to your body.

Medical Solutions

There are methods of Hormone Replacement Therapy (HRT) that some women find particularly helpful. For some women, these methods may not have as much of an impact or may have the opposite impact. Every woman has different levels of hormones in her system. Some women may have higher levels of testosterone in their system, others may have levels of estrogen that fluctuate more frequently. What other options exist out there for women?

Consider the Impact of Phytoestrogens

Phytoestrogens are naturally occurring compounds found in plants that bind to cells just as estrogen does, only at a weaker affinity. Many women are hesitant to consider phytoestrogens as a form of treatment, but there are some benefits to taking phytoestrogens, especially when it comes to sex drive. However, some researchers have found that phytoestrogens in certain compounds may be able to help increase sex drive.

Phytoestrogens from plants and plant compounds like maca, fennel, and maritime pine bark have been observed to improve sexual function.

Conditions like dyspareunia, experiencing vaginal pain during sexual intercourse, were also found to decrease slightly after using these specific ingredients. Phytoestrogens from the fenugreek plant, specifically, were shown to have some positive effects on libido. Fenugreek is largely cultivated in India. Consider using supplements that have these plant compounds to help alleviate issues with low libido or other sexual health issues.

ॐ

Mood swings may feel like they're out of your control, but that isn't necessarily true. There are steps you can take to better regulate your moods by decreasing their intensity and frequency

ॐ

Chapter 3 - Mood Swings

As women, we're all too familiar with mood swings. From the moment puberty begins, our hormones rage war on us. One cute animal video can make us burst into ten minutes of tears on any given day during our menstrual cycle. Other days we may feel easily irritated. Some days we may feel angry and lash out at others without provocation.

Vanessa's Story

I have a partner who is understanding and incredibly supportive. We've been married for 24 years. He is my best friend, constant companion, and I love him more than anything. But even that didn't stop the menopause monster inside me.

A few years ago, I found myself saying hurtful, insensitive and downright cruel things to him. This was most decidedly not normal, and when I started digging into what might be causing it, I made sure to include him in my research process. I reported back the things my healthcare provider told me about menopause and its effect on mood, and how it can cause irritability to the point of seeming irrational. It was important to me that my husband know that he was not the cause for all the anger and combativeness I was feeling.

Could he be irritating, and did I get genuinely angry about things? Of course. No human is perfect, and no relationship is all roses and romance. But making sure that he knew what was causing this change in me, and what he could do to help me, was one of the primary ways in which I made my menopause journey better for both of us.

I encourage women to actively engage their partners in conversations about menopause as soon as they feel they may be approaching it. The changes that perimenopause and menopause can bring to a woman can and do affect her entire family. The more you can share, openly and honestly, the stronger your relationship can become.

While we may have coping mechanisms to deal with mood swings during menses, mood swings during perimenopause can be especially challenging. The intensity and frequency of mood swings change as we go through perimenopause.

How Does Menopause Affect Mood Swings?

When perimenopause begins, the two primary sex hormones, estrogen, and progesterone begin to drop. These hormones are not just responsible for regulating sex organs. They also have an impact on other hormones, specifically neurotransmitters, that regulate mood and emotional responses. Estrogen helps facilitate the synthesis of serotonin, a neurotransmitter that contributes to feelings like happiness, content, and pleasure along with dopamine. When estrogen levels fluctuate, serotonin levels are also impacted. When estrogen levels are high, serotonin synthesis and production tend to increase. When estrogen levels are low, serotonin production also lowers.

There are obviously multiple factors that can contribute to mood stability and mental health that are individual to every woman. Women who have been diagnosed with clinical depression, anxiety, bipolar disorder, and so on will have other hormonal and chemical factors that contribute to their moods. In order to better understand how certain mental health conditions or neurological disorders may be affecting your moods during menopause, speak to a licensed healthcare professional who specialized in those areas to get the best care possible.

What Moods Do Mood Swings Encompass?

Mood swings can encompass any kind of emotion. The key is recognizing how abruptly your mood changes from one thing to the next, especially if those moods distinctly contrast each other. Of course, the most common moods are similar to those that women may feel during their menstrual cycle. If you were to experience one of these moods one minute and a completely different mood the next, chances are you're experiencing mood swings. This is especially prevalent for women in perimenopause.

This includes:

- Irritability
- Unusual Weepiness
- Anxiety
- Excitement
- Depression

Mood swings may feel like they're out of your control, but that isn't necessarily true. There are steps you can take to better regulate your moods by decreasing their intensity and frequency.

Diet

Diet impacts your brain as much as it impacts your heart, bones, and all the other systems in your body. While there are some studies that show certain foods can have a temporary impact on dopamine levels, there's more to adjusting your diet in menopause than just eating "feel-good" foods. Eating foods with specific nutrients, vitamins, and minerals can help improve your brain health and better regulate mood.

What kinds of foods are beneficial to regulating mood? For women in menopause, consuming moderate amounts of foods with phytoestrogens can help to slightly improve hormonal imbalances and moderate mood. What are phytoestrogens?

Phytoestrogens are compounds that naturally occur in plants. They act similarly to the estrogen your body produces, just at a weaker level.

Research is still being conducted about the impacts of consuming large amounts of phytoestrogens, as they can have some negative effects in regards to other medical conditions and interact with certain medications. However, it is generally thought that a moderate intake of phytoestrogens can provide some health benefits.

What kinds of foods contain phytoestrogens?
- Soy products like tofu, tempeh, soymilk, and miso
- Vegetables like cauliflower, broccoli, brussel sprouts, and cabbage
- Fruits like plums, cranberries, strawberries, and raspberries
- Seeds like flax seeds and sesame seeds

Exercise

One of the best ways to improve mood is to exercise on a regular basis. Exercise has a fountain of benefits that are not just associated with weight loss. Engaging in exercise can boost your immune health, cardiovascular health, muscle health, bone health, and most importantly, brain health. Just how exactly can exercise help improve your mood?

When you exercise, your body naturally increases its production of endorphins. Endorphins are neurotransmitters that reduce our body's perception of pain and can make us feel calm or produce pleasure. So, how does an increase in endorphins help stabilize mood or prevent intense mood swings? The primary culprit that triggers mood swings is stress. Stress hormones, primarily cortisol, can cause different receptors in the brain to behave abnormally. By increasing endorphins you can actually lower cortisol levels and lower overall stress, allowing your brain to synthesize and release serotonin, dopamine, and other neurotransmitters.

So what kinds of exercise should women in menopause engage in? How often should they exercise? How can women adjust exercise routines to better reflect their needs and their overall comfort?

The Power of Moderate-Intensity Exercise

What does the term moderate-intensity exercise mean? As women we hear this term thrown around so often as a way to improve weight loss but how many of us know what it actually means? Moderate-intensity exercises are forms of exercise that get you moving fast enough to burn off 3 to 6 times more energy per minute than you would sitting down, but without adding extra strain to your body like intense muscle aches or joint pain.

Moderate-intensity exercises tend to be low-impact exercises that help strengthen cardiovascular health. However, there are ways to incorporate other types of exercise into a moderate-intensity workout regimen that can address other physical health concerns like bone health and muscle health. Weight-lifting and resistance exercises can be categorized underneath moderate-intensity exercises depending on how much strain you're putting on your body. What are some moderate- intensity exercises? Let's break it down into some categories.

Cardio and Aerobic: Cardiovascular exercises are exercises that increase your heart rate. Aerobic exercises are exercises that require your body to use oxygen at a higher amount than you would standing still. Both of these exercise categories often encompass the same kinds of exercises because when your body begins to use more oxygen it increases your heart rate.

So, some common cardio and aerobic exercise include:

- Jogging
- Brisk Walking
- Swimming
- Cycling
- Dancing

Weight Lifting and Resistance: Menopausal women are highly encouraged to start incorporating weight lifting exercises, or lower impact resistance exercises into their routine. Why? Weight lifting and resistance exercises have a number of health benefits that could reduce the risk of developing certain conditions, mainly osteoporosis. How do these exercises help reduce the risk of developing osteoporosis? Well, when you engage in any kind of strength training, you encourage the synthesis of new bone tissues to form. When this happens your bone density begins to increase and it reduces the risk of fractures.

Some excellent weight lifting and resistance exercises include:

- Walking with light-weight dumbbells
- Pilates with light resistance bands (things like pelvic presses and single-leg stretches)
- Beginner weight-lifting exercises like curls and chest presses (start off with light weights and work your way up from there, but make sure to keep the weight at a comfortable amount without too much strain)

Interval Training: Many athletes at the professional level use this method to train for competitive events, marathons and so on; but did you know that interval training could be a viable exercise option for you? Interval training is a type of training that involves alternating between different activities at different speeds and different degrees of effort/exertion. Let's look at some examples to get the full picture.

Walk at a comfortable pace for 1-3 minutes, then switch to a jog or sprint for 30 seconds. Take a 1-minute rest, also known as a recovery and then repeat the process.

Do jumping jacks for 1 minute and then take a 30 second resting period, then go back to jumping jacks.

By alternating between increasing heart rate with a high-intensity exercise and lowering your heart rate through a recovery period, you are actually encouraging your body to become more relaxed after each resting period, which could help better stabilize your mood as your metabolism rate can last longer even after you've finished a workout.

There are plenty of options for you to choose from when it comes to exercise. Pick regimens that you feel comfortable with and most of all, listen to your body. If something doesn't feel right or feels like it's putting too much strain on joints or muscles, readjust your exercise plan. You may feel that your exercise routine will come down to a lot of trial and error at the beginning, but don't be discouraged. You will find what's right for you.

Stress-Relief Management

Ultimately mood swings come down to a change in hormone levels. Now, this change can be brought on by any combination of factors from dropping estrogen levels to mental health conditions. However, the biggest contributing culprit is stress. Natural hormone fluctuations are enough of a challenge to combat on their own, but when you add increased stress to the mix, that struggle is compounded.

Women of menopausal age often experience high amounts of stress. Family stress, work stress, financial stress, even social stress can all exacerbate menopausal symptoms and have a significant impact on both your mental and physical health. Stress hormones like adrenaline and cortisol can exacerbate mood swings, especially in high-stress situations like a busy day at the office or heated arguments with family members.

Managing stress may seem easier said than done but there are ways in which women can better manage their stress in their daily lives, even if it's only for a few minutes. What are some ways that you can use to better manage your stress?

Breathing Exercises

Before you throw in the towel and resign yourself to stress becoming your new normal, consider this. Breathing exercises do have an impact on stress levels, they may be fairly temporary but they do work. How? Stress triggers our body's natural fight or flight response, which in essence is a basic survival instinct that helps us identify and combat danger, or rather, what our mind perceives as dangerous.

When stress is high, your breathing patterns change, and your heart rate increases. You'll begin to take shorter, shallower breaths as your lungs attempt to distribute oxygen-rich blood to your body more quickly which, in turn, will increase your heart rate in an effort to pump blood more quickly.

So, how do deep breathing exercises help combat this problem? When you take in a deep breath, your brain registers it as a sign of relaxation and sends signals to the rest of the body that it needs to relax, ultimately lowering cortisol and adrenaline levels. Your muscles will relax, your heart rate will become steady, and your lungs will be able to increase the oxygen levels in your blood without added strain.

Alright, enough with the scientific explanations, let's get down to what you want to know. If you feel stressed and you need to do some deep breathing exercises, what should you do?

Dr. Andrew Weil developed a deep-breathing strategy that draws inspiration from the yogic technique called pranayama. If you're familiar with this technique then this should be easy to integrate into your routine. This breathing technique is called the 4-7-8 deep breathing exercise. It's intended to help relax the mind and the body by forcing both to focus solely on your breathing. So, how does it work? First, find a comfortable position, either sitting or laying down. Next, make sure to empty your lungs of any air you may have taken in previously. Once you're ready, begin by inhaling through your nose for a count of 4 seconds. Next, hold that breath in for a 7-second count, if you need to place your hands on your abdomen to make sure your diaphragm is steady. Finally, pursing your lips to make a whooshing sound, exhale that breath in a steady stream for 8 seconds. If your hands are placed on your abdomen, make sure not to put added pressure on it as you feel your diaphragm lower. Repeat this process up to four times.

By using this technique, you can help lower your heart rate and prepare your body for a state of relaxation. When this happens, your cortisol levels will drop and your body will be better able to stabilize your moods.

Build a Support Ecosystem

There's an important distinction to make between a support ecosystem and a support network. A support network is described as the group or groups of individuals that provide you with support, comfort, and advice as you combat a particular problem, which makes it a part of the support ecosystem.

The support ecosystem is the environment that you immerse yourself in as a way to receive the support, comfort, and advice you require to combat a problem. This includes having family, friends, and other individuals to talk to about certain problems. This also includes how you implement changes in order to overcome a struggle, whether it's through the influence of a specific atmosphere or how you seek out solutions (like talking to a therapist or joining a support group).

The real question is, how do you go about building a support ecosystem that works for you? Not every woman is going to require the same elements to make her support ecosystem work for her. So, where do you start in building a support ecosystem that's right for you?

First, identify what you value most. Do you value comfort from friends and family? If yes, then you should make strides to keep those relationships strong and to have open communication with the. Do you feel you would benefit from having the insight of other women in menopause? Then joining a support group of women in menopause may provide that for you. Do you feel you would benefit from some alone time and personal reflection about your experience before you are ready to discuss them with someone else? Then take an hour out of your day to dedicate to some personal reflection, whether it's writing thoughts and feelings down or just working out your frustrations on an evening jog.

Second, develop coping mechanisms that work for you when you start to feel overwhelmed. Some women find comfort in channeling their stress into a creative outlet, be it painting, sewing, writing. Others will take a few minutes to get up and get the blood flowing when they feel stressed. Whatever helps you stay calm and stay motivated to complete daily tasks should be implemented in your routine.

Talk to a Therapist

When all else fails and you still feel your mood swings are taking control of you rather than you are of them, talk to a therapist. There could be some deeper issues that your mind is actively repressing and a therapist can help guide you to overcome those issues. Your mood swings may also be affected by more than just your menopause or stress, they may be affected by a mental health condition that you were previously unaware of. A therapist may be able to help point you in the right direction and recommend you to a medical health professional that can help you come to a diagnosis and get you on the right track for treatment.

Supplements

Research into how supplemental ingredients affect mood has produced some interesting findings. While herbal, mineral, and vitamin-centric remedies are not cure-alls for menopausal symptoms, they can provide some relief so long as they are taken consistently and used correctly. You might be wondering, how can a supplement help regulate mood? Well, it's important to understand how certain compounds might have an impact on your brain.

Vitamin B6
Vitamin B6 also referred to as pyridoxine, is coenzyme consisting of six compounds that helps facilitate several functions within your body. Most importantly, it's been found to play a critical role in brain health. How so? Vitamin B6 can help increase the production of the neurotransmitters serotonin, dopamine, and gamma-aminobutyric acid (GABA). All of these neurotransmitters help regulate mood and can increase feelings of calm, happiness, and pleasure. Vitamin B6 has also been found to have some impact on decreasing levels of the amino acid homocysteine in the blood. Research has found an interesting correlation between high levels of homocysteine and increases in depression, which suggests that there might be a link between the two.

It's important to note that your body cannot produce Vitamin B6. You have to obtain it through foods or supplements.

ॐ

Irregular periods are usually
the first noticed sign of
perimenopause in women.

ॐ

Chapter 4 - Changing Periods

Changes in periods are not a strange phenomenon for women. From the moment we hit puberty, we've often felt like our periods had minds of their own. Sometimes they're early and decide to stain that pair of pants we've been itching to try out. Sometimes they're so late we go out and buy pregnancy tests only to see that little negative symbol turn up after 3 minutes of waiting. Sometimes they come with debilitating cramps. Sometimes we only feel a mild amount of fatigue but a lot of bloating. They're light, they're heavy and then light again.

Regular periods may not be something many of us are accustomed to at first, but once they do become regular, it feels like a blessing. It means no more guessing games, no more surprise visits from Aunt Flow, and a consistent list of menstrual cycle symptoms. So what happens when that regular period cycle we were overjoyed to receive starts to teeter off and become irregular again?

The stress and frustration of irregular periods during perimenopause can be immense. Some women who may have never experienced menstrual headaches before are now suddenly bombarded with multiple headaches on the first day of their period. Maybe your menstrual cycle used to last 4 days, now it lasts up to 8. Instead of 3 weeks between periods, you might experience 2 periods in a month.

Vanessa's Story

A few years ago, I had a period that lasted for 3 weeks. All my life, I have been incredibly regular when it comes to my cycle, so needless to say, I was pretty worried.

And this wasn't just three weeks of mild bleeding. It was 21 days of bleeding through super-ultra-mega-could-absorb-the-Pacific-Ocean tampons. Twenty-one days of cramps, bloating, and none of my clothes fitting. Twenty-one days of worry, stalking forums, and online research.

A visit to my gynecologist confirmed it: perimenopause.

I've since learned that periods in perimenopause can be wildly fluctuating realities for many women. I've even spoken with several women who've told me that they didn't have a period for 2 entire years, and then had one!

The more we can do to regulate the fluctuations of our hormones, the better we can address things that can accompany it, like wildly unpredictable periods. Read on for some of the steps you can take to help regulate your periods, and better understand what is causing them in the first place.

Irregular periods are usually the first noticed sign of perimenopause in women. They could be attributed to other factors like stress or a change in diet, but more often than not when periods start to be consistently inconsistent, it means perimenopause has arrived.

What Do We Mean by Irregular Periods?

How do you know if your period is irregular? What if you're someone who normally isn't regular? When we talk about irregular periods we're talking about a number of different issues. Not every woman experiences periods the same way so how could they know if they're experiencing irregularity? There are a few common traits of irregular periods that women have cited over the years that can help you determine if you're experiencing an irregular period cycle.

Changes in Period Duration
Changes to the time your period lasts can be a sign of irregular periods. Under a regular cycle, your period might usually last around 4 or 5 days. Once perimenopause starts, you might be experiencing periods that last 6, 7, 8 days. Some women have even reported their periods lasting up to 2 weeks!

Changes in Period Frequency
Not only can a period's duration change, but you can also experience changes to your menstrual cycle's frequency. Your period may be earlier or later than usual. Some women have even had 2 periods in a month. If your period arrives a day or two before it's supposed to on the calendar, you might have nothing to worry about. However, if your period is four days or even a week early, then it could be a sign of perimenopause.

Changes in Period Symptoms
Noticing an early period or two may not be the only way to identify whether you're experiencing perimenopausal-related irregular periods. Your menstrual symptoms can change too. Experiencing more headaches could be a sign of irregular periods. Having more intense cramps or increased fatigue could be a sign of irregular periods. Whatever symptoms you don't experience normally during a period should be taken into account before you come to any conclusions. If you're unsure about whether certain symptoms are normal for you or not, speak to a doctor and perhaps you two can come to a more solid conclusion.

What Causes Periods to Change?

Estrogen and progesterone levels don't drastically decrease the moment your body senses it's time for perimenopause to begin. Hormones will begin fluctuating before they start decreasing. This means that you could have a sharp surge of hormones that cause your period to behave strangely before they finally begin to lower over time. This fluctuation of hormones can last from a few months to about a year or possibly two years for some women. Hormonal fluctuations are normal to experience but they can be especially frustrating when keeping track of periods, as women in perimenopause can still become pregnant.

How Can Irregular Periods Impact Your Health?

Irregular periods can be frustrating, but more than that, they can have a great impact on your health. For some women the changes to their periods cause them to have abnormally heavy flows. They may even bleed through super-absorbent tampons or pads. In some cases, women who have abnormally heavy periods during perimenopause can develop anemia due to the large blood loss.

Anemia is a condition in which a person does not have enough healthy red blood cells to carry oxygen throughout the body. This may cause some women to feel dizzy when standing or sitting during their menstrual cycle. It may also increase feelings of fatigue both on and off your period. Oftentimes women who are anemic also suffer from an iron deficiency, which can impact how quickly your body produces red blood cells.

Irregular periods can also have an impact on your sleep patterns. Many women who experience increased cramps or headaches on their periods have increased trouble falling asleep and staying asleep. This causes them to wake up periodically throughout the night and unable to fall asleep for long periods of time. Without proper sleep, your body's overall ability to function decreases. Sleep helps properly regulate the immune system. It helps your brain synthesize information and store memories. It helps your muscles relax and repair themselves, especially after a workout.

It doesn't stop there, irregular periods could also affect your mental health. Your hormones play a role in regulating mood. When those hormones are constantly fluctuating, they can affect what kind of moods you experience both in their intensity and their frequency. Some perimenopausal women have reported feeling increasingly depressed or anxious during and well after their menstrual cycles.

Why You Should Discuss Irregular Periods With Your Doctor

You may not think irregular periods are having a negative impact on your health, but you'll never know for certain unless you talk to your doctor. Talking to a licensed OB/GYN can help you better understand how your body is impacted by irregular periods. If you're not sure where to start when talking to your OBY/GYN about your concerns, here are a few questions to keep in mind.

1. Based on what I've described, what could be going on?
2. Are there treatments available to me based on the issues we've addressed?
3. What are those treatments?

4. What are some of the side effects of those treatments?
5. What are some lifestyle changes I can make to alleviate some of these problems?
6. Should I complete any additional tests?
7. What are those tests and what do they do?

Being proactive about your health during perimenopause will make it that much easier for you and your doctor to find the best course of action for you and help you find the right treatment. So be honest and don't be afraid to ask questions.

What Are Your Treatment Options?

Not all women experience irregular periods in the same way, which means that not all treatments are going to work equally for women in perimenopause across the board. There are a variety of treatment options out there, but finding the right one can be a bit tricky. Some of the more common treatments include hormone replacement therapy options, over-the-counter medications, lifestyle changes (adjustments to diet and exercise), antidepressants in some cases, as well as herbs and supplements.

How Can Supplements Help?

Some combinations of supplemental ingredients have helped to alleviate some premenstrual issues in young women and women of perimenopausal age. These ingredients tend to include Vitamin B6, calcium, manganese, and so on. How can all of these ingredients help alleviate period problems? Well, they can be used to treat a variety of issues.

Vitamin B6

Vitamin B6 is primarily used to help improve mood and reduce depression. Vitamin B6 helps synthesize and regulate major mood-stabilizing neurotransmitters, particularly serotonin, dopamine, and gamma-aminobutyric acid (GABA). Because of this, PMS symptoms like increased irritability, anxiety, and depression often decrease. A three-month study of 60 perimenopausal women showed that by taking 50 mg of Vitamin B6 on a daily basis, nearly 69% of the participants felt a decrease in PMS moods like irritability, depression, and anxiety.

Vitamin B6 has also been thought to help prevent and treat anemia. Vitamin B6 has some role in the production of hemoglobin, which is what red-blood cells need in order to circulate oxygen throughout the body.

ॐ

A common symptom in
menopause, as well as a
source of extreme frustration,
is the change to bodyweight.

ॐ

Chapter 5 - Weight Gain

A common symptom in menopause, as well as a source of extreme frustration, is the change to bodyweight. Women tend to experience weight gain more often than weight loss during the stages of menopause, although both can occur depending on a series of factors. Weight gain is not only a serious health concern for many women, but it can also impact self-confidence for women in mid-life.

Vanessa's Story

Ah, weight. It's something I have struggled with my whole life: from being underweight in my early twenties as I danced 8 hours a day, to being morbidly obese by the time I was in my early thirties. I've been able to shed 40 pounds in my forties, but it is a constant struggle to keep it off.

The second I eat sugars or fried foods, my microbiome is thrown out of whack, and I have to battle to get it back in balance. Those unhealthy bacteria can really take a foothold in my gut! I am so glad I discovered that the microbiome plays such a huge role in weight gain, because I feel like I finally have the tools to manage my weight.

Now it is up to me to keep the fried food and sugar off my plate. It's not always easy, especially around the holidays, but knowing that keeping my microbiome healthy helps me manage my weight definitely makes it easier to do, and that makes all the difference.

According to The National Health and Nutrition Examination Survey, 68.1 percent of women between the ages of 48 and 59 were classified as overweight or affected by obesity, whereas 51.7 percent of women between the ages of 20 and 39 were classified as overweight or affected by obesity. That's a 16.4 percent increase within a difference of about 20 years. This also shows how weight gain issues tend to occur most often during the perimenopausal years. What causes such a significant increase in weight gain for women in their menopausal years?

Weight Gain in Menopause: How Does It Happen?

We've seen that estrogen can have a laundry list of effects on the female body.

It impacts everything from hormones to bones to brain health and much, much more. So, how does it impact body weight? A form of estrogen known as estradiol helps regulate metabolism and body weight in women.

When estradiol levels are low, the body increases its number of stores fat in the body. In the younger adult years, it's not uncommon for women to carry most of their weight in their hips and thighs. Once women enter perimenopause, that weight will start to shift more towards the abdominal region. The fat in this area is called visceral fat. It's the fat that is stored between your vital organs and the membrane of your abdominal cavity and it can work its way into your arteries if you aren't careful.

This kind of fat is especially dangerous. Why? Well, unlike the subcutaneous fat (the fat that lies directly underneath the skin), this fat can affect several areas of the body. Visceral fat produces hormones and substances that can increase blood pressure, increase insulin resistance which makes it more difficult for your body to use insulin effectively, cause inflammation, increase the risk of developing certain cancers, and contribute to sexual health problems.

It seems like there are a lot of hurdles to get over already. You may have thought that weight loss was difficult enough as a younger woman, but now with the lowering levels of estrogen, it might seem almost impossible to you. Don't worry, it's not impossible. There are ways to help you achieve your weight loss goals even in menopause.

Healthy Weight Starts with Healthy Habits

You've heard it from every licensed healthcare professional, personal trainer, and gym rat alike, "The key to weight loss is a healthy routine of diet and exercise."

Well, we hate to play the captain obvious card, but they're right. The first step in your weight loss program should be adjusting aspects of your lifestyle, starting with diet and exercise.

Now, by and large, we understand that many women lead hectic lives. Working a 9 to 5 job, coming home to take care of family, social engagements, maybe even some of you do community and charity work on a regular basis. We get it, being busy means you need a quick fix to some of the smaller things. This means skipping out on the exercise and ordering takeout from that Chinese place just down the street.

Convenience comes with consequences and like most people, you may not pay attention to those consequences at first but over time you will begin to see how they impact you. Diet and exercise don't just impact your weight. They impact the health of your immune system, the health of your brain, the health of your bones, and your heart. The health benefits to a proper diet and regular exercise are practically endless. Of course, you may have eaten well and exercised regularly during your younger years but you're still seeing areas of weight gain.

What do you do then?

There are ways menopausal women can adjust their diet and exercise routines to better reflect their needs both as women in menopause and as individuals with personal health issues.

What Does A Balanced Diet Look Like in Menopause?

Women in menopause have slightly different dietary needs than younger women, younger men, and men of similar ages. calories depending on how active they are. Obviously, the individual woman may have certain dietary needs based on her own medical history or genetics. So these guidelines should be adjusted according to those specific needs.

Dairy
Dairy products are full of necessary nutrients that maintain proper bone health like calcium, phosphorus, potassium, magnesium, vitamin D, and vitamin K. During menopause, women are at higher risk of developing osteoporosis due to the loss of estrogen. To combat this, it's suggested that women in menopause find ways to increase their calcium intake. It's fairly easy to do this with dairy products as foods like milk, cheese, and yogurt tend to have higher quantities of these key nutrients.

However, not all women can eat dairy products. In fact, between 30 and 50 million people in the United States are lactose intolerant, many of whom are women. This puts these women at higher risk of developing osteoporosis and even experiencing perimenopause earlier than the average (non-lactose intolerant) woman. Let's look at some of the foods that are rich in these nutrients for both lactose intolerant and non-lactose intolerant women.

Foods High in Calcium (this is just a small sample of a whole host of calcium-rich food options!)

- Milk
- Cheese
- Yogurt
- Leafy Greens
- Tofu
- Fortified beverages
- Soymilk
- Salmon
- Lentils

Whole Grains

Whole grain products are important to menopausal health mostly due to two things fiber and B vitamins. High fiber diets have been linked to a reduced risk of developing heart disease, certain cancers, and in some cases premature deaths. While many people think they are consuming enough fiber in their current diet, more often than not, people consume refined grains rather than whole grains.

What's the difference? Whole grains are grains that have nutrients from their 3 main parts: the bran, the endosperm, and the germ. Refined grains tend to only have the endosperm intact, which means you're only getting 1/3 of the nutrients you need. An example of a refined grain is white bread. White bread is refined white flour, which means nutrients from

the bran and the germ have been milled (stripped) from the grain.

Whole Grain-Rich Foods
- Whole Wheat Bread
- Brown Rice
- Quinoa
- Rye Bread
- Oats
- Corn

Fruits and Vegetables
Fruits and vegetables have the most variety of essential nutrients, vitamins, minerals, and fibers that the body needs. This is why American dietary guidelines tend to suggest that you fill half of a plate with fruits and vegetables at every meal. You might think that eating a banana a day or a small bowl of mixed berries might be enough to satisfy your body's fiber requirements or antioxidant needs.

However, only 14% of American adults reported eating at least 2 servings of fruit and 3 servings of vegetables daily in 2009. If the percentages were that low then, how far have those percentages come in the ten years since then?

There is an abundance of benefits to adding more fruits and vegetables into your diet. First, they can provide you with antioxidants and other nutrients to help promote a healthy immune system. Second, many of them are rich in fiber. Fiber is essential to help people with their weight loss goals. Why?

Dietary fiber helps your body expel waste more efficiently by helping increase the size, weight, and softness of stool. Why is this important to weight loss? Well, as women age, their bodies start to hold on to larger quantities of waste. By increasing your fiber intake, you're actually helping your body process waste more efficiently. Fiber helps improve your liver function, keeping it from becoming dehydrated and slow. Fiber also acts as an appetite suppressant, meaning that if you consume large enough quantities of it it will help you stay full for longer and less likely to feel hungry. This means that you won't go searching for those sugary treats to snack on during your weight loss journey.

Fruits and Vegetables to Incorporate

- Apples
- Bananas
- Raspberries
- Strawberries
- Artichokes
- Beets
- Broccoli
- Carrots

Protein

The bones are not the only area of the body that are affected by a decrease in estrogen. Muscle mass also decreases in women as they go through menopause. For women trying to lose weight or trying to get in shape, this can make things especially difficult as your muscles are the primary protectors of your bones.

Ensuring your muscles are healthy can also help you as you progress in your workouts, and good quality protein is the key to helping muscles stay healthy.

Women in menopause are encouraged to consume higher quantities of menopause. In fact, women over 50 are suggested to consume 0.45-0.55 grams of protein per pound of your body weight as part of your daily value in comparison to the daily recommended 0.36 grams per pound for young adults over 18. Not only can this help them from losing muscle mass, but it can also help you feel less hungry by decreasing the levels of hormones responsible for triggering hunger responses.

Foods High in Protein

- Eggs
- Lentils
- Fish (All Types, but Tuna is one of the highest)
- Meats (Pork, Chicken, Lean Beef)
- Asparagus
- Shrimp
- Quinoa
- Peanuts

Diet is Half the Battle, Exercise is the Other Half

Changing diet is often the easier part of the weight loss battle. Yet, for most people, implementing a regular exercise routine is the difficult part. Changing or starting an exercise routine can be difficult for several reasons. Finding time to set aside for a good workout can be tricky, especially if you work non-stop 9-5. Figuring out what kind of workout routine you should try is another hurdle. With so many workout programs and types of exercise out there, it can be difficult to find the right routine for you. If gyms and personal trainers make you feel uncomfortable, it can be hard to find the motivation to exercise on your own.

Starting and sticking to an exercise regimen requires a lot of decisions, and that can be a bit daunting. Don't panic, there are steps you can take to help you out and get you started on the path to fitness fast.

Step 1: Decide What Workout Environment Works Best

Deciding how you're going to work out is the first big step. Some people thrive in a public space, and the local gym helps them to feel motivated, as well as learn helpful techniques to better their workout goals. Some people feel more comfortable in a private setting and working out in their own home helps them stay focused. Some people need outside motivation to help them stay on track, in which case a personal trainer is best for them.

How do you know which workout environment will work best for you? Here are a few questions to keep in mind to help you identify your ideal workout environment.

1. How comfortable would you feel working out in front of other people on a scale of 1 to 10, 1 being the least comfortable and 10 being the most comfortable?
2. Are you more motivated by setting goals on your own or are you more motivated to have someone else set goals for you and help you get there?
3. Do you want to use your workout time as a way to make friends or see existing friends?

Write down your answers on a piece of paper before you go onto the next step, and be honest.

Step 2: Decide How Much Time You Will Dedicate to Exercise

Your schedule may only allow you to have a small, finite amount of time to dedicate to exercise, and that's okay! The key to deciding how much time you'll dedicate to exercise is identifying how much time you have and if you're willing to make room for more time if you need it. It's recommended that people get at least 20 minutes of moderate to vigorous exercise in a day, but if all you can squeeze in is 5 minutes of light exercise here and there then segment out your time so you can do it multiple times in a day.

If you're thinking of rearranging your schedule to incorporate your workouts, keep these questions in mind.

1. How much time a day do I spend at my work or my home life?
2. How much free-time do I have in a week?
3. How long would I like to workout?
4. What time of day would I like to workout?
5. What time of day do I feel the most tired?
6. What time of day do I feel the most awake?

Step 3: Decide What Workouts You Want to Try

Deciding what kinds of exercise you want to try out can be the most daunting part of the process. There are 100s of different workout programs out there for you to choose from, and thousands of exercises you can incorporate into your daily routine. How do you pair everything down to a manageable list of options? You'll have to make a series of mini decisions here.

1. What problem areas are you trying to address?
2. What is your current exercise routine regiment like? Has it been working for you?
3. Do you experience things like joint pain when doing simple things like sitting or standing?
4. What exercises do you enjoy or think you would enjoy (i.e. dancing, swimming, pilates, weight lifting)?
5. What exercises do you want to avoid or think you would not enjoy (i.e. kickboxing, crossfit, running, biking)?
6. Have you had any past injuries or surgeries? If so, where?

Step 4: Come Up With a Basic Plan

Once you've answered some of these questions and you have a rough idea of how you're going to start your new exercise routine, do a little research and come up with a basic plan that you think will work for you. If you decide you want to try lifting weights at a local gym with the help of an instructor or personal trainer, determine how you're going to get there. Find a gym you like and sign up for a membership you feel comfortable paying for. See what instructors or personal trainers work with that gym and choose which one you want to work with.

Maybe you're planning on working out from home and want to purchase the least amount of equipment possible so you choose a pilates workout routine. Fantastic! Now's your time to plan things out. Decide when you're going to workout at home, how long you're going to workout for, what videos or online classes you're going to try out, and if you choose, how you're going to decorate your workout area at home.

Once you've got a basic idea of how you're going to implement your workout routine into your life, it's time to move onto the next step and the last hurdle.

Step 5: Follow Through and Adjust

This is it! The moment you've been waiting for! You've got everything planned out! You've made sure to square out your schedule! Now it's time to get to that workout. Now there are one of 2 ways this can go. Your first workout under this new routine can work out very well for you. You might find it's exactly what you need to get on the track to fitness.

On the other hand, it could turn out that it doesn't fit your needs at all. Whether it doesn't fit your schedule, the exercises seem like they're too easy or too difficult for you, or you feel uncomfortable in your workout environment; find out what areas are giving you problems and readjust your plan. There's nothing wrong with deciding something isn't working out and moving on to something different. Just be sure to identify what isn't working out and take all the necessary steps to fix it.

Can Supplements Come to the Rescue?

You might be familiar with the promise of weight loss supplements that populate the market and you might think they're a complete hoax. Well, to some extent you're right. There are products on the market that will promise to boost your metabolism so high that you'll shed 5 pounds a day, and you should be wary of them. However, there are supplemental products that can help you with your weight loss goals by providing additional assistance to your weight loss routine; a routine that should consist of a healthy diet and daily exercise.

That being said, there are probiotic supplements that can help aid with the weight loss process. You might be wondering, how in the world can a probiotic help me lose weight? Well, probiotics can do a number of different things for your body, and one of them is to help improve your body's natural metabolism.

The real question is, what probiotic ingredients are best suited to help the weight loss process along?

Lactobacillus Gasseri

Lactobacillus gasseri (l. gasseri) is a strain of lactobacillus that can help with fat distribution. As women age into menopause, the body begins to distribute fat to the abdominal region, often in the form of visceral fat. Lactobacillus gasseri helps reduce fat distribution to the abdominal region. By reducing fat

distribution to this area, the overall percentage of fat stored in this region begins to decrease as there is less adipose tissue (fat) to store energy from food into.

Lactobacillus Plantarum

Another strain of lactobacillus that can be beneficial for weight loss is lactobacillus plantarum (l. plantarum). Lactobacillus plantarum's effects can help you maintain a healthy weight in a number of ways. First, l. plantarum can aid in the reduction of glucose levels in the blood. When blood glucose levels are high, the risk of increasing weight gain and developing diabetes increases.

Additionally, l. plantarum can help maintain intestinal permeability. Intestinal permeability is the body's ability to control the passing of material (primarily nutrients) from inside the gastrointestinal tract, through the lining of the gut, and help it spread throughout the body. By regulating intestinal permeability, your body is better able to extract nutrients from food.

Bifidobacterium Animalis-B420

One of the many challenges to maintaining weight loss is not giving into hunger. The stomach naturally produces a substance called Ghrelin. When Ghrelin passes through the microbiome and enters the brain, it stimulates certain receptors in the brain that results in feeling hungry. Bifidobacterium animalis (B. animalis) is a strain of bacteria that permeates through the microbiome and helps suppress feelings of hunger. How does it do this? Studies have shown that one strain of B. animalis, ssp. Lactis 420, increases and balances the production of serotonin, one of the neurotransmitters responsible for mood regulation. However, serotonin also functions as an appetite suppressant. It curbs feelings of hunger and lowers activity in the brain caused by Ghrelin.

If You Have Questions, Speak to Your Doctor

For the many women of menopausal age who are diabetic or have additional health issues that need to be specifically addressed during the weight loss process, we strongly recommend that you speak to your doctor/general care provider about those concerns. You may have underlying health conditions you didn't know you had that are affecting your metabolism and your ability to lose weight. Always, always, always speak to a doctor about any concerns you have before you start making adjustments to your diet, your exercise routine, and your medications.

౸

When we talk about menopausal insomnia, imbalances in hormones are primarily responsible for disrupting the body's natural sleep cycle.

౸

Chapter 6 - Insomnia

How many of you can relate to this scenario?

It's 7:30 at night, you've had one of the most stressful days at work in the history of your career. You come home, put your feet up, maybe pour yourself a nightcap, and spend the evening watching your favorite show. You look at the clock and see how late it's getting. You feel exhausted from today so you go about your night routine and clock out for the night around 10 o'clock. You think you'll fall fast asleep, after all, your day has been a nightmare. Instead, you're lying awake in bed thinking about all of the things you have to get done tomorrow that you didn't get around to today.

You can't turn your brain off! Your mind fixates itself on that spreadsheet you forgot to put together for your boss or the fact that you've forgotten to call your sister for the fifth time in a row this month. You finally drift off to sleep around 11:30. You think you'll be able to sleep through the night with no problems.

Then surprise! You wake up for no reason at all. You bolt up in bed and look at the clock. It's three in the morning. You can't fall back asleep. You try everything. You get a glass of water from the kitchen. You try tuckering yourself out by staying up and watching a show or movie that used to put you out like a light. You try to see if sleeping on the couch will be more comfortable. Finally, your body wills itself to sleep around 5:30 maybe six in the morning, and you have to be up at seven. Your alarm goes off at 7 o'clock sharp. You feel more tired than you did yesterday, but you have to push through it and get out of bed.

The first thing you feel, apart from exhaustion, is a headache, then maybe a neck ache. Your joints are stiff. Your muscles are somehow sore. You wonder how that could be since you did nothing but sit at your desk all day yesterday. You feel annoyed, agitated, and no amount of coffee in the world will save you from how tired you are. You can't concentrate. You mess up making coffee four times in a row. You burned your breakfast. You missed the sink after brushing your teeth and toothpaste is now stuck to the toe of your shoe. You think to yourself, "This is not my morning."

If this describes how most of your nights are spent, then you're probably experiencing one of the most dreaded menopausal symptoms, insomnia. One in four women will have some insomnia symptoms in their lifetime and about one in seven adults suffers from chronic (long-term) insomnia.

What is insomnia? Insomnia is a sleep condition that can interfere with your body's natural circadian rhythm. People with insomnia tend to have difficulty falling asleep, staying asleep, and wake up periodically throughout the night. This condition can impact everything from your immune system to your metabolism to your memory.

What Causes Insomnia in General?

There are plenty of factors that can affect sleep patterns and increase insomnia. However, when we talk about menopausal insomnia, imbalances in hormones are primarily responsible for disrupting the body's natural sleep cycle. How would a hormonal imbalance cause insomnia, you ask? Let's take a closer look.

The Relationship Between Estrogen and Melatonin

We've talked a lot about how estrogen affects the body, and yes it extends far beyond regulating the sex organs. We know it can impact bone health, muscle mass, and so on, but did you know that it can impact your sleep too? Estrogen has a close working relationship with its friend, melatonin, the hormone responsible for inducing sleep. When estrogen levels are low, melatonin cannot be synthesized as quickly. This means it can take longer for you to fall asleep.

Why Women Can't Turn Their Brains Off at Night

You've probably heard or used this phrase when describing sleep problems. You lay in bed, hoping to drift off to sleep but you can't seem to tell your brain to stop talking. Your thoughts are buzzing around in your head and they're somehow so loud that you can't calm your brain down enough to fall asleep. You might think this is just a phenomenon you create for yourself, but there is a science behind it.

One of the primary neurotransmitters in the human body is gamma-aminobutyric acid (GABA). Of the many roles that GABA plays in the human body, one of the most important is its role in inducing sleep by helping the brain and the body relax. GABA helps regulate the activity of neurons. When neuron activity is high, you naturally feel more awake. When neuron activity is low, you feel more relaxed and it becomes easier to sleep. So, when GABA is properly regulated it binds to neurons and reduces their activity. When this happens, information transmitted to the brain from neurons throughout the nervous system is inhibited, causing you to feel calmer and allowing your body to prepare for sleep.

Why is Sleep Important in Menopause?

Sleep is important for the human body regardless of age or health status, but it is especially important to get a good night's sleep during menopause. As we age, our ability to retain memory is greatly affected. One way to combat extreme cases of memory loss is to get enough sleep. There's a state in our sleep cycles called Rapid Eye Movement (REM) sleep. REM sleep is the deepest stage of sleep when the eyes move back and forth rapidly underneath the eyelid. Now, how does REM sleep improve memory? When we experience REM sleep, our minds are able to process, synthesize, and store information in our brains more effectively. Without REM sleep we would be unable to store and retrieve memories.

Why should this concern you as a menopausal woman?

According to the Alzheimer's Association, two-thirds of Americans living with Alzheimer's are women. Women in their 60s are two times more likely to develop Alzheimer's than breast cancer and of the 5 million people in the United States who are diagnosed with Alzheimer's, 3.6 million of them are women. That's more than half of the total population of people with Alzheimer's disease.

So we can agree it's good for your memory if you get a good night's sleep, but what else can sleep do for you? Getting enough sleep can help keep your immune system strong, repair muscle tissue, and help heal blood vessels and tissue cells that make up your heart. Ongoing sleep deprivation can lead to increasing the risk of developing serious illnesses like heart disease, kidney disease, high blood pressure, and even stroke.

How Can You Improve Your Sleep?

Dealing with sleep deprivation is frustrating. You may have tried everything you can think of, from changing out your pillows to switching the sheets, to sleeping with a white noise machine on in the background. Making changes to your sleeping environment is one solution. There are other things you can do to help you sleep better at night.

Make Some Changes to Your Diet

We've talked a lot about the gut-brain axis and the power of the microbiome, but did you know that your gut could also be impacting your sleep? There are two areas of the body that have the largest concentration of neurons, the brain, and the gut. There are around 100 million neurons in your brain, all sending and receiving information. There are 500 million neurons in your gut, scientifically known as the gastrointestinal enteric nervous system. That's five times the amount of neurons in your brain! The term "gut-feeling" might have more scientific merit than you think. So, how can you take better care of your gut?

Cut Down on Caffeine

You may already be familiar with this tip, but it's important to understand why so many doctors tell women in menopause to cut down their caffeine intake. Caffeine is a substance known as a stimulant, meaning it helps increase neuron activity.

When neurons fire rapidly, the brain's overall nervous activity remains high, which means that both the brain and the body are in a hyperactive state and cannot relax.

You may think that those few cups, or pots, of coffee in the morning and during the workday have little effect on you when you're ready to go to bed but that's not necessarily true. Obviously, everyone metabolizes caffeine a bit differently, but on average it takes between 4 to 6 hours for caffeine to make its way through your body and eventually wear off. So if you drink two 6-ounce cups of coffee, it could take anywhere from 12 to 14 hours for that caffeine to wear off.

If you drink enough coffee in a day to take over 12 hours to wear off, then your sleep cycle will be completely thrown off. Your neurons will be in a hyperactive state and your body won't be able to reduce that activity as effectively.

Eat Sleepy Foods

When we talk about sleepy foods, we're talking about foods that can provide your body with sleep-inducing compounds. It may sound like some strange kind of magic at first, but trust us, there are foods out there that can help you feel sleepy. What kinds of foods can help you fall asleep?

Turkey

Not only is turkey an excellent source of nutrients, as well as absolutely delicious, but it also contains an amino acid that can help you feel sleepy. The amino acid tryptophan can help boost the production of neurotransmitters like the sleep inducer melatonin and the mood regulator serotonin.

Almonds & Walnuts
Another interesting sleep aid is the chemical element magnesium. Magnesium stimulates and helps regulate your parasympathetic nervous system, which helps your body relax and prepare for sleep. Magnesium also helps regulate melatonin and it binds to GABA receptors, which as we know help turn your brain off by reducing neuron activity. While very few women may be magnesium deficient, around 75% of people in the U.S. don't get enough magnesium in their diet. Almonds and walnuts are great sources of magnesium. In fact, one ounce of almonds can provide you with 19% of your daily value of magnesium.

Fatty Fish
Fatty fishes like salmon, tuna, trout, and mackerel are known for their health properties. These fishes are rich in omega-3 fatty acids and are good sources of vitamin D. Both of these can help improve your heart health and bone health, but did you know that these two nutrients can help you fall asleep? When combined, omega-3 fatty acids and vitamin D can help increase serotonin production. Serotonin, another neurotransmitter, acts as a mood stabilizer making you feel calm and happy. Higher levels of serotonin can help you relax and prepare your body for sleep. So, next time you eat sushi, make sure to keep the fatty fishes coming.

Passionflower Tea
Passionflower tea has been used to treat a variety of health issues for many years. It's been used to treat anxiety, to boost immune health, and to reduce the risk of heart disease. However, its sleep-aid properties are what make it fascinating. Passionflower contains an antioxidant known as

apigenin. This antioxidant helps create a calming effect throughout the brain by binding to certain receptors, primarily GABA receptors. This means that passionflower tea may help reduce the activity of neurons and help both the brain and the body to fall asleep faster.

There are plenty of other foods out there that have been looked into for their sleep properties. We recommend you speak to your doctor or a licensed nutritionist to get a complete list of sleep-aid foods.

Change Your Bedtime Habits

We're not just talking about switching out pillows, mattresses, and sheets. When you think of your bedtime habits, think of what you would normally do before you go to sleep. You've brushed your teeth, washed your face, and so on, but what else do you do before bed? Do you watch TV? Do you check your emails on your phone? Do you watch 30-second videos of cute animals?

Using electronic devices before bed can actually do more harm than good. You may think you're just engaging in a mind-numbing activity to help you fall asleep, but in reality, you're exacerbating the problem. Electronic devices (mobile phones, tablets, laptop computers, TV screens) emit an artificial blue light that can inhibit sleep.

Blue light suppresses melatonin production and without adequate levels of melatonin, your body cannot relax and prepare for sleep. Blue light can delay the process of falling asleep twice as much as other forms of light. It can alter your body's natural circadian rhythm and it can even keep your body temperature elevated, which can make it more difficult to fall asleep, as well as make it easier to experience hot flashes at night.

So, rather than turn on the TV or spend time checking emails on your phone, set a timer to stop using those devices before bed. It's recommended that you stop using electronic devices between 30 minutes and an hour before you go to bed.

Are You A Sensitive Sleeper?

Sometimes your sleep environment affects you in different ways. You might be someone who gets cold easily at night. You might be someone who has sensitive skin and certain fabrics can be irritating. However, the most common types of sleep sensitivity are sound and light sensitivity, especially for women. Because your body has a more difficult time regulating sleep hormones and neurotransmitters, your body is automatically more sensitive to elements in your sleep environment that seem distracting.

How to Combat Light and Sound Sensitivity

If you find you need complete silence when you're about to go to sleep or you need the room to be pitch black, there are ways that you can help create that environment to minimize the number of distractions before you fall asleep. Unplug devices that create high-pitched white noise before you go to bed. Put up blackout curtains in your bedroom. Put small pieces of dark tape over electronics that have small lights, especially LEDs. Sleep with an eye mask on, to keep any excess light from outside disturbing you.

I've Tried Everything! Now, What Do I Do?

Let's say you've tried changing your diet. You've cut out caffeine. You started eating turkey before bed. You've made changes to your environment. You put up blackout curtains and unplugged that alarm clock that seems to make an endless buzzing noise. You're still having trouble falling asleep, or if it's not falling asleep, it's staying asleep. So, now what? What can you do to find some relief?

Consider Using Supplements

There are a variety of supplemental ingredients available to women that can offer some relief for women with insomnia. Herbal ingredients, vitamins, and minerals, as well as some probiotic strains, can help balance your microbiome. When your microbiome is healthy, your gut-brain axis can improve your body's ability to regulate hormones, neural activity, and overall health. So what supplements and supplemental ingredients should you consider before you talk to your doctor about treatments?

L-Theanine
L-Theanine has become a popular treatment option for a number of reasons. The most important to note is that l-theanine has been shown to help reduce anxiety and provide stress relief. It helped lower cortisol levels and reduced heart rate, both of which are ideal conditions for sleep preparation. By helping lower the heart rate and reducing cortisol levels, the body becomes relaxed, which can help trigger the brain to increase melatonin production and begin the sleep process.

Vitamin D3
There is a complex interplay between estrogen and vitamin D. Levels of vitamin D decline with age and people with vitamin D deficiencies are more likely to suffer from insomnia and other sleep conditions. Although the relationship between vitamin D and sleep quality has not been precisely pin-pointed there are a number of

connections to suggest a strong relationship between the two. Every cell in the human body has some kind of vitamin D receptor including neurons in the brain and, more specifically, the hypothalamus. This means that when vitamin D enters the body, through food or through sunlight, cells in the hypothalamus bind to that vitamin D and regulate a whole host of bodily functions, most importantly, sleep. The loss of estrogen, coupled with vitamin deficiencies that occur in menopause, can disrupt sleep.

Magnolia Bark Extract
Magnolia bark extract has been used as a sleep aid for thousands of years in some eastern cultures. Why? Magnolia bark acts as a sedative in many ways due to the presence of two major polyphenols, honokiol and magnolol. Some studies have found that introducing small quantities of magnolia bark extract reduced the time it took for subjects to fall asleep. Additionally, like l-theanine, magnolia bark acts as a stress-reliever. By lowering cortisol levels in the body, magnolia bark extract can help the body feel calm. By lowering the heart rate, the body is better prepared to begin the sleep process.

What Have We Learned?

Insomnia and other sleep conditions can affect our health in multiple ways.

It can make us more prone to developing illnesses, make it more difficult to maintain memory, and affect our ability to focus even when completing simple tasks. However, there are a variety of solutions you can implement in your daily life to reduce the severity of insomnia. Focus on balancing the microbiome through food and supplements, and eliminating distractions before bedtime.

ॐ

You are not alone.

ॐ

Conclusion - You Are the Master of Your Menopause

As women in menopause, we are constantly bombarded with negativity, disbelief, and skepticism from others. We try to find sympathy and support, but often there is a disconnect between us and our support network. We cannot truly explain everything we experience in menopause and expect 100 percent of the people we speak to entirely understand. This can be extremely discouraging for a lot of women, as they feel they have no way to move forward and take charge of their menopausal journey if others are unwilling to listen.

It's up to us as women to be proactive, to break down barriers, and to facilitate the conversation in the right direction. That can seem like a daunting task, but with the right tools, we can make progress and bring the attention that menopausal health needs.

Managing your menopausal journey can seem overwhelming but with the right resources and the right mindset, you may be surprised at how quickly you get comfortable with it. The key things to remember are these:

Be Open About Your Needs

Whether it's talking to your doctor, your partner, your friends, or your kids, being open about your needs as you go through menopause is crucial to maintaining your relationships and your overall health. Speak to your doctor about your health concerns and work with them to get the treatment you need and maintain long- lasting health. Speak to your family about the changes you need to make in your lifestyle to make sure your menopausal experience is the happiest and healthiest it can be. This should encompass diet changes, lifestyle changes, and maintaining healthy communication with family members. Speak to your friends about your social withdrawal or anxieties. Let them know that your mental health is being affected and that you're taking the steps you need to improve it.

Be Proactive About Your Health

At the end of the day, you are the only one who can promote and maintain your health. If you don't take charge of your health or your health concerns, no one else is going to make the effort. Being proactive about your health means taking action. Make changes to your diet, your exercise routine, and adjust areas of your lifestyle based on your needs. Implement systems that work for you that you can continue with ease.

Ask Questions and Gain Knowledge

Don't be afraid to ask questions because as we all know, knowledge is power. If you're curious about something, be it medications, supplements, meditation, or nutrition, ask your doctor. Ask for the professional opinion of healthcare workers, experts, and researchers. Don't worry about being perceived as bothersome or annoying. Medical professionals are there to help you identify your health problems and help you treat them so that you can live life to the fullest.

Remember You're Not Alone

Above all, remember that you're not alone in your menopausal concerns and experiences. Turn to other women for advice, insight, and support. There is a whole community of women out there who are going through similar struggles and their support can be just as important for you to have. Join support groups, apps, forums, and community groups. Find your tribe and support each other. And remember that the entire team at MenoLabs is here to support you.

Visit us at MenoLabs.com

References

We'd like to recognize the organizations, researchers, and medical publications that have made these incredible strides in menopausal research. It is through their hard work that we were able to create this book. We strongly encourage readers to look through these research studies, not only to gain a better understanding of menopausal health, but also to recognize the dedication of these medical researchers.

Chapter 1: Hot Flashes

Dietz BM, Hajirahimkhan A, Dunlap TL, Bolton JL. Botanicals and Their Bioactive Phytochemicals for Women's Health. *Pharmacol Rev.* 2016;68(4):1026-1073. doi:10.1124/pr.115.010843

Ehsanpour S, Salehi K, Zolfaghari B, Bakhtiari S. The effects of red clover on quality of life in post-menopausal women. *Iran J Nurs Midwifery Res.* 2012;17(1):34-40. Retrieved from https://www.ncbi.nlm.nih.gov/pmc/articles/PMC3590693/

Hidalgo LA, Chedraui PA, Morocho N, Ross S, San Miguel G. The effect of red clover isoflavones on menopausal symptoms, lipids and vaginal cytology in menopausal women: a randomized, double-blind, placebo-controlled study.

Gynecol Endocrinol. 2005;21(5):257-264. doi:10.1080/09513590500361192

Rosedale R, Westman EC, Konhilas JP. Clinical Experience of a Diet Designed to Reduce Aging. *J Appl Res.* 2009;9(4):159-165.

Retrieved from https://www.ncbi.nlm.nih.gov/pmc/articles/PMC2831640/

Rotem C, Kaplan B. Phyto-Female Complex for the relief of hot flushes, night sweats and quality of sleep: randomized, controlled, double-blind pilot study. *Gynecol Endocrinol.* 2007;23(2):117-122. doi:10.1080/09513590701200900

Introduction to Menopause. *Johns Hopkins Medicine.* Retrieved from https://www.hopkinsmedicine.org/health/conditions-and-diseases/introduction-to-menopause

Chapter 2: Low Sex Drive

Najaf Najafi M, Ghazanfarpour M. Effect of phytoestrogens on sexual function in menopausal women: a systematic review and meta-analysis. *Climacteric.* 2018;21(5):437-445. doi:10.1080/13697137.2018.1472566

Naumova I, Castelo-Branco C. Current treatment options for postmenopausal vaginal atrophy. *Int J Womens Health.* 2018;10:387-395. Published 2018 Jul 31. doi:10.2147/IJWH.S158913

Palma F, Xholli A, Cagnacci A; as the writing group of the AGATA study. The most bothersome symptom of vaginal atrophy: Evidence from the observational AGATA study. *Maturitas.* 2018;108:18-23. doi:10.1016/j.maturitas.2017.11.007

Chapter 3: Mood Swings

Hartvig P, Lindner KJ, Bjurling P, Laengstrom B, Tedroff J. Pyridoxine effect on synthesis rate of serotonin in the monkey brain measured with positron emission tomography. *J Neural Transm Gen Sect*. 1995;102(2):91-97. doi:10.1007/BF01276505

Hvas AM, Juul S, Bech P, Nexø E. Vitamin B6 level is associated with symptoms of depression. *Psychother Psychosom*. 2004;73(6):340-343. doi:10.1159/000080386

Mikawa Y, Mizobuchi S, Egi M, Morita K. Low serum concentrations of vitamin B6 and iron are related to panic attack and hyperventilation attack.

Acta Med Okayama. 2013;67(2):99-104. doi:10.18926/AMO/49668

Chapter 4: Changing Periods

Doll H, Brown S, Thurston A, Vessey M. Pyridoxine (vitamin B6) and the premenstrual syndrome: a randomized crossover trial. *J R Coll Gen Pract*. 1989;39(326):364-368.

Retrieved from https://pubmed.ncbi.nlm.nih.gov/2558186/

Chapter 5: Weight Gain

Barreto FM, Colado Simão AN, Morimoto HK, Batisti Lozovoy MA, Dichi I, Helena da Silva Miglioranza L. Beneficial effects of Lactobacillus plantarum on glycemia and homocysteine levels in postmenopausal women with metabolic syndrome. *Nutrition*. 2014;30(7-8):939-942. doi:10.1016/j.nut.2013.12.004

Cerdó T, García-Santos JA, G Bermúdez M, Campoy C. The Role of Probiotics and Prebiotics in the Prevention and Treatment of Obesity. *Nutrients.* 2019;11(3):635. Published 2019 Mar 15. doi:10.3390/nu11030635

Hosterman JF. The Truth About Menopause and Weight Gain. Obesity Action Coalition. 2014. Retrieved from https://www.obesityaction.org/community/article-library/

the-truth-about-menopause-and-weight-gain/

Strus M, Chmielarczyk A, Kochan P, et al. Studies on the effects of probiotic Lactobacillus mixture given orally on vaginal and rectal colonization and on parameters of vaginal health in women with intermediate vaginal flora. *Eur J Obstet Gynecol Reprod Biol.* 2012;163(2):210-215. doi:10.1016/j.ejogrb.2012.05.001

Vásquez A, Jakobsson T, Ahrné S, Forsum U, Molin G. Vaginal lactobacillus flora of healthy Swedish women. *J Clin Microbiol.* 2002;40(8):2746-2749. doi:10.1128/jcm.40.8.2746-2749.2002

Zhang R, Daroczy K, Xiao B, Yu L, Chen R, Liao Q. Qualitative and semiquantitative analysis of Lactobacillus species in the vaginas of healthy fertile and postmenopausal Chinese women. *J Med Microbiol.* 2012;61(Pt 5):729-739. doi:10.1099/jmm.0.038687-0

Appendix 2. Estimated Calorie Needs per Day, by Age, Sex, and Physical Activity Level. 2015. Retrieved from https://health.gov/our-work/food- nutrition/2015-2020-dietary-guidelines/guidelines/appendix-2/

State Indicator Report on Fruits and Vegetables. Centers for Disease Control and Prevention. 2009. Retrieved from https://fruitsandveggies.org/stories/ adults-and-adolescents-arent-eating-enough-fruits-and-vegetables/

Chapter 6: Insomnia

Chen CR, Zhou XZ, Luo YJ, Huang ZL, Urade Y, Qu WM. Magnolol, a major

bioactive constituent of the bark of Magnolia officinalis, induces sleep via the benzodiazepine site of GABA(A) receptor in mice. *Neuropharmacology.* 2012;63(6):1191-1199. doi:10.1016/j.neuropharm.2012.06.031

Gao Q, Kou T, Zhuang B, Ren Y, Dong X, Wang Q. The Association between Vitamin D Deficiency and Sleep Disorders: A Systematic Review and Meta-Analysis. *Nutrients.* 2018;10(10):1395. Published 2018 Oct 1. doi:10.3390/nu10101395

Gottesmann C. GABA mechanisms and sleep. *Neuroscience.* 2002;111(2):231-239. doi:10.1016/s0306-4522(02)00034-9

Nobre AC, Rao A, Owen GN. L-Theanine, a natural constituent in tea, and its effect on mental state. *Asia Pacific Journal of Clinical Nutrition.* 2008;17 (S1): 167-168. Retrieved from http://apjcn.nhri.org.tw/server/APJCN/17%20Suppl%201/167.pdf Ritsner M, Miodownik C, Ratner Y, Shleifer T, Mar M, Pintov L,& Lerner V L-Theanine Relieves Positive, Activation, and Anxiety Symptoms in Patients With Schizophrenia and Schizoaffective Disorder: An 8-Week, Randomized, Double-Blind, Placebo-Controlled, 2-Center Study. Published 2010 Nov 30. Retrieved May 26, 2020, from
https://www.psychiatrist.com/JCP/article/Pages/2011/v

72n01/v72n0105.aspx Siegel JM. The neurotransmitters of sleep. *J Clin Psychiatry*. 2004;65

Suppl 16:4-7. Retrieved from https://pubmed.ncbi.nlm.nih.gov/15575797/ Williams J, Kellett J, Roach P, Mckune A, Mellor D, Thomas J,& Naumovski N. L-Theanine as a Functional Food Additive: Its Role in Disease Prevention and Health Promotion. *Beverages, 2*(2), 13. Published 2016. doi:10.3390/beverages2020013